Cracking

Cracking Up

My Experiences of Schizophrenia

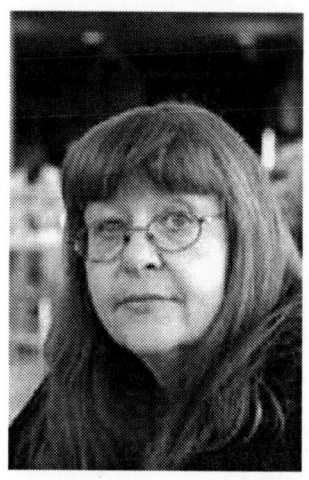

By Deirdre Geraghty

One million people commit suicide every year.
The World Health Organization

Cracking up & Barkin'

All rights reserved, no part of this publication may be reproduced by any means, electronic, mechanical photocopying, documentary, film or in any other format without prior written permission of the publisher.

>Published by
>Chipmunkapublishing
>PO Box 6872
>Brentwood
>Essex CM13 1ZT
>United Kingdom

http://www.chipmunkapublishing.com

Photographer Eric Hands

Copyright © Deirdre Geraghty 2007

Cracking up & Barkin'

To my son Philip, who has grown into a kind and thoughtful
person with a wonderful sense of humour.

To my friends who did their best to stand by me along the way and all
who supported me.

With a special thanks to Dr. Richard Wales.

Cracking up & Barkin'

Cracking up & Barkin'

Since a young child, I'd always planned my children – I'd have them first as it was all I could think about – and when they were safely off my hands then would be time to study for a career. Children were the most important thing to me – teach them at home – take them to the swings and the museums and the library. At least two, one was unkind.

The week I fell pregnant (after eight years of waiting), my husband lost his job. He had been there eight years and was a Junior Director of the Company. It was a total shock, not only had he lost his job but we lost a large part of our social life as well.

When Philip was one, I was being told to go back to work. I wouldn't listen, blank it out, I couldn't be parted from my child, I must be calm – I must be strong.

When Philip was two, the Bank Manager said I must return to work or lose the flat. I was heartbroken; I couldn't believe I was to be parted from my son. Although it was only supposed to be for a few months, just to get a little money in.

And then it started....

My first day there and I was told by the others in the office that my job used to be done by two people and I should say that it is too much for one. It was a challenge and I quite enjoyed it but leaving Philip was so upsetting. I just wanted to

Cracking up & Barkin'

get through this with as little pain as possible. I was told not to talk to the girl in the corner as nobody spoke to her and very soon they stopped speaking to me as well.

The harder I worked the angrier they became. Caroline in the corner and I became friends but then she was moved to another office so I was on my own with them. We met for lunch each day and shared our experiences of the others which helped.

And so it continued. I was getting up at 8.00. Getting Philip ready for nursery which was heartbreaking; doing a day's work in silence, meeting Philip at 5.30, going to the playground ("The Swings,") making his tea, putting him to bed with a story at 9.00 when I would nod off. Then up again to cook the dinner, share a smoke (cannabis), boil up water to do all the washing by hand (we had no washing machine, hot water nor heating). Fall into bed by 1.00 AM by which time Philip would get up as he had been asleep at the nursery in the afternoon and would want to learn to read or other such activity until I could stay awake no longer. Then, of course, I had to be up again by 8.00.

Day in...day out...week in...week out. The girls in the office becoming worse and worse. Being 'sent to Coventry' wasn't very pleasant. I would go out to lunch and they would be celebrating a birthday when I returned and I was never included.

Cracking up & Barkin'

I had never experienced anything like this before. I was so tired but I must be calm and I must be strong.

This went on for nearly a year. I was distraught. Being separated from Philip all day for a year was so distressing but we made up for it half the night. The strain was enormous yet all the way through I had a strong feeling that as long as I remained calm and strong for Philip then he would be okay. Yet remaining calm and strong was the hardest thing.

I started to wonder why I was married and what about more children? I could barely cope with getting up and getting to work now. I was like a zombie, at the end of my tether but at least Philip was fine.

Then I got a crush on a man at work. We went out for a drink and then a meal. I moved into the spare room. And then everything went haywire. The gossiping and the whispering got a whole lot worse. The guy at work stopped talking to me, "I was a married woman with a child".

I 'phoned a Solicitor to discuss Divorce, at least I would get single parent benefit and tax relief. I might as well be on my own with Philip. I mean, what is the point of a husband who is never there, is not much help and no support either financially or emotionally. I was going through all this at work and no prospect of more children. I need a better partner, one who would care for me and my child. But the thought of divorce came hard to me. A strong Catholic upbringing, I had never considered this outcome.

Things started to happen. My husband started whispering with his friend. They would giggle over the 'phone and he told me about the girl he fancied in the Baker shop. He would go to the pub after work and play darts and leave me to it.

Things started to happen at work. People started to be behaving strangely. And my head started to feel like an over-used switchboard. As though all the lines were busy and calls waiting. I could feel, almost hear all the thought of the others around me. I could feel them all thinking about me. As though they were directing thoughts towards me, pushing me, testing me. Can I cope? Of course I will cope, I thought. I must be strong. I will pass this test. I thought I must be telepathic as I can hear all these thoughts being directed towards me.

My husband seemed to be doing the same thing. They must all be in it together. What's going on? I have never experienced anything like this before but I have to keep this job and my home if I am going to bring up the child on my own. Everything seemed to turn into tasks, I felt I had to pass all sorts of tests and then I would no longer be an outsider.....I would be included, accepted. No longer put through all of this. I just had to remain calm and strong and work out what was going on and all this would stop.

Cracking up & Barkin'

Caroline went on holiday. So I went home for lunch, had a quick bite. Maybe if I have a joint it will help me. Not that I put much in as I wasn't used to rolling my own. It might take some of the pain away as the girls in the office had abandoned any restraint now Caroline was away.

I had to go the Store Room. There was apparently an ancient well down there in the basement. The old caretaker warned me I would get into trouble if I went down there... what did he mean?
And then one of the girls in the office spoke to me, could she borrow a hat for Ascot. I lent her one but couldn't understand what was going on. And then it came to me.... it's witchcraft.... she's after a hair from the hat. They're casting spells on me.... that is what's going on.... that's why I feel so strange....

And then my husband gave me a doll, a wooden doll, with strange wide awake eyes and I realised that I was no longer sleeping. They were all in it together. Definitely witchcraft. But why? And what was I to do. I started to get terribly frightened. I could feel their thoughts all around me. And the guy in the office, he seemed to hate me even more than the girls. And the more he stormed through the office, the more the girls whispered and banged the furniture to make me jump when I walked past.

Then one morning I went into work and everything had changed. One of the girls was

Cracking up & Barkin'

sitting at my desk, on my 'phone, with my files, doing my job. I've failed the test, I thought. I'll fight, I won't let them fail me, I have a child to support. I remembered the tune I had heard the night before. As I had lain awake for another night I had heard the tune. I had wondered where it was coming from. I thought it was some kind of message coming from the guy at work who seemed to be next door.... what does it mean? Perhaps if I sing that tune, that row of notes, they will realise I'm on the right track. I'm not going to fail this test.

I put the voodoo doll on the desk and started to sing that tune, over and over again. And then I was called into my Boss' office. Could he help? Would I like to see a Doctor? "No" I said "I need a priest". So they took me and the wooden doll to the priest. I hadn't seen a priest in a very long time but felt a little relieved that he had taken charge of the staring object. And when I told him of the witchcraft at work and that my husband was involved he suggested a Doctor.

So I was taken to the Doctor. But my Doctor wasn't there... what had happened to my Doctor..... who was this man sitting at his desk.... and why was his 'phone off the receiver... somebody is listening at the other end. What is going on? "You're sick" he said "I'm not" I thought. They might like me to think I am but I know I'm not. I was delivered home with a bottle of tablets, my son taken to my sister. My husband smiling ' Take your tablets and have a nice weekend with your husband and you will be okay" I was told.

Cracking up & Barkin'

I could hear them, hundreds of them, outside in their cars. And my neighbours... they had all gone out, the houses dark, nobody home. What is going on? Don't like this.... why had my Boss wanted to see my tablets. Of course, it's a pharmaceuticals company, they want to overdose me... kill me.... good job I hadn't let him see. If I hide the tablets they won't know what to give me. Bottom of the toy box, they'll never look there.

I lay in the marital bed and my husband coming down on me... the look of glee in his eyes and suddenly he looked evil... I can't bear this... I run in to the spare room and sit, terrified, feeling their presence outside. Why were they doing this? What was going on? I need to get help... I'll go to Westminster Cathedral tomorrow. They'll know what to do. They know all about witchcraft. I'll be safe there, they'll get help. They'll work out what's going on.

The next day I put on my running shoes; put money in my pockets and at first light head for the bus. I can feel their presence all around me and see that look in the eyes of those on the bus, jump off and onto another. More of them, jump off the bus and run. The sun comes out... God is with me... the clouds cover it and the others are winning. Into the safety of the Cathedral. I find the vestry and the priest there says he's heard about me from my local priest. I said they are trying to

Cracking up & Barkin'

kill me and he said "what right had I to question God, when it is my time to die I must accept it". Then he prayed over me and was gone.

Terrified out of my mind I meet an old nun. I had always felt safe with the nuns at school and she looked kindly. "Go to the Jesuits" she said "they're clever; they'll know what to do". So I got a bus and headed into town. I could feel danger all around me and when I was told by the Jesuit to stop talking nonsense and surround myself with good people and be on my way I didn't know what to do. I found myself in Oxford Street. I kept seeing those wearing crosses... God was winning and then I would see those horns people wear and people with Nike on their T-shirts (that stood for 'Old Nick' – the Devil) and I thought "I'm losing". What should I do?

I found solace with the tramps... they had kindly faces. There was one on the corner by Oxford Circus Tube, blind he had said, selling matches, would I get him a coffee. He whispered reassuring words and then, directed by a Policeman, I headed for the Hare Krishna place in search of food. I knew I would be safe if I surrounded myself with a lot of people but there were few there and all the food was gone. There was a young man who said he knew where we could go in the country where there were lots of people. We got a tube and then a bus when I realised he had ulterior motives. We had just passed Walthamstow Tube... I didn't know where we were going. It wasn't safe. I quickly jumped off

Cracking up & Barkin'

the bus and ran back towards the tube. I rang the Police "please help me", I said, "stay where you are and we'll come and get you". I thought they might look like ordinary police but who knows and where will they take me. And then I saw them... the people from Oxford Street... that look in their eyes... I had to get away... I ran down the escalator and onto a tube. But it didn't move... "Please hurry or they will catch up", I thought. So I blessed myself with the Lourdes water and Rosary I had been given at the Cathedral. The woman opposite looking quite uncomfortable.

Where can I go? I sat the whole distance on the train and got off at Brixton. I know, I thought, I'll go to the Police Station...."They're trying to kill me", I said "they're involved in witchcraft, my husband's involved". I'll take you to a safe place" he said "I'm walking that way" and he took me to a Christian commune. It felt like a safe house and they gave me a cheese sandwich whilst they quoted from the Bible. They told me I couldn't stay there but if I walked home I would be perfectly safe, put my faith in God. So off I set through Brixton to Clapham and through the common. It was about 1.00 on Sunday morning but the journey was peaceful and nobody bothered me.

My husband was still up but said nothing about the day. He would take me to church in the morning but not the Catholic Church; we would compromise and go to Holy Trinity, the "Church of England" church set up by William Wilberforce on the common. I slept like a baby.

Cracking up & Barkin'

So off we went to Church (I hadn't been for years). It was a bright sunny morning. And there they all were... all the people from yesterday. Smiling at the two of us... with a look of knowing on their faces. Who are they? What were they up to? Obviously pleased to see us together. All the way to the Church... more and more of them... grinning faces. I can't go in there... I ran towards the Catholic Church my husband running after me. But they were there as well, setting up their market stalls to sell their plastic statues... Jesus would smash them if he were here. They looked at me with their grinning faces. I ran back to the commune where they were praying in 'tongues'. But to them that meant in French and Spanish... this isn't the place to get help, where should I go? I ran and jumped on a bus, feeling their presence all around me. They mustn't know where I'm going, if I am to get help I have to get there before them. Not knowing where I was going I jumped off the bus and ran.

It was August Bank Holiday and all the good people were leaving London for the country. Two of the guys at work had been joking about hunting... they liked to hunt. That's what this was... it was a hunt and I was the prey. All the good people leave town and they have a hunt every year. I came upon the Queen's Cavalry or whatever they were, opposite Rochester Row Police Station. "Tell the Queen" I thought. But I couldn't find the way in. So I stumbled into the

Cracking up & Barkin'

Police Station. "What are you going to do", I asked the Policeman. He burst out laughing "nothing" he said.

I ran and ran and found myself outside Westminster Abbey. A vicar in the forecourt gave me the address of a convent in the East End. So with the aid of my tube map, I arrived there as quickly as possible. Hiding... running... escaping. There must be help somewhere.

The Order of St. Margaret. "Help" I said "I need sanctuary". They let me in and made me a bowl of porridge as I hadn't eaten all day. They removed my tube map and 'phoned my elder sister. It was quite late by this time but they took me by car to the local mental hospital.

"Have you smoked cannabis" she said amongst other things and "we'll put you in the blue ward". I lay there clutching the rosary for protection. What were they after? I thought of my child. A very special little boy and realised that was it... he hadn't been christened, he was very clever and very sensitive and very deep. They wanted him. They wanted to kill me and gain control of my son. My husband was weak and had joined them, there was no protection there. What was I to do? But in order to get the child they had to get rid of me. At least they couldn't get to me in here. I had to stay awake in case they got in during the night but I could rest. The man watching me from the end of the bed, with his light pointing towards me, was disturbing but he couldn't let them in if I stayed awake.

Cracking up & Barkin'

The next day I was accompanied to breakfast and in for various 'chats'. Apparently, I was on suicide watch. I had said my death would look like suicide. As long as I was here Philip was safe and when I left I would go into a convent. They will never get me there and I can get help.

In the afternoon I was ushered into a sitting room and there they all were. People from the tube and Oxford Street. The same people over and over, watching me, grinning at me and here they were visiting my fellow patients. They were all connected. I wasn't safe at all. I have to get out of here, out of London. I have to remain safe or they will get my child.

My Mum and sister visited me the next day. My sister was accused of supplying me with cannabis. She was totally shocked. What was this Doctor talking about? She knew nothing about cannabis. It was arranged for my child to go to Mum in Kent and me to be transferred to a hospital nearby. It would be safe there.

A car was arranged. I was to be accompanied to Kent. The man travelling with me couldn't find my file and was told it had been filed in the bin. They have binned me, I thought. And then I saw the driver of the car, he was very old, I was amazed he could still drive... and then it hit me, it would be a car crash; I was to die on the way. My chaperone announced he was getting out along the way and I thought that then I would die... I won't let him get out; if he stays in the car I'll get

Cracking up & Barkin'

there. The lorries either side on this motorway were huge and fast and very close and I prayed with all my heart all the way there. The journey seeming fraught with danger of one sort or another.

They put my things on the bed in the corner. I'm not going to be trapped in the corner, I thought, so I look for an empty bed in the middle of the ward and move my things there. There seems to be some sort of confusion as to who my Doctor is, some sort of panic at my arrival, they mustn't put my husband down as my next of kin as I don't trust him and he will let them give me electric shock treatment. My sister, I'll give her name instead.

I could feel more of them approaching outside. They were listening to everything I said through the open window with some kind of listening device. The air felt electric. "Why do you think you feel this way?" I was asked "Perhaps they put something in my coffee" I said. "Why would they?" he said. "I would love to think this is an illness" I said, "but I know it's not, I know it's real"

I sat up all night, enclosed by the curtain around the bed, clutching my belt and a shoe as my only forms of defence, listening to the two nurses. It was as though everything they said related to me. It was as though they were talking on one level about their own lives but there were messages on a different level which were meant for me.

Cracking up & Barkin'

As the days went past I realised that these messages were all around me, on the radio and the television and in everything that people said. Like a parallel universe. They were talking about one thing but everything they said reinforced the things that I was thinking. I checked the wiring to the television, the pipes that ran around the building wondering how it was being done. I wondered if there was something in the cigarettes being smoked – or the smoke itself. On one day I would be closing all the windows to stop people outside listening to what I was saying or even thinking, on another I would be opening them to let the smoke out. Sometimes the staff would laugh at me or despair at what I was doing next.

And me gripped by an absolute terror at what I perceived going on around me. I had listened to the screams in the night of what I though was the very fat lady. I thought that she was being barbecued alive, that once you found yourself in one of these places there was no escape, you would be fattened up by the food and the medication and nobody would believe you; a sudden suicide or two, who would notice?

I realised these things were going on all over England and that the patients were in terrible danger so it was down to me to get help. Where could I take them? Perhaps there was a convent nearby which would take us in. I had to get into the office to find a map or a phone book. I talked with the other patients. "I have always known I was different" said one. I have too. I realised there

Cracking up & Barkin'

was something different about all of us. Are we Psychic? What is it about us that we are different?

Realising the futility of my plan to take all the patients to somewhere of safety, I decide that it is down to me to go and get help.

Where am I to go? Perhaps Rome, to see the Pope? Escape to France and hitch across Europe. Not possible. No, I must get to Ireland. I'm pretty sure these things don't go on there. There is a programme on the telly about boats. Another message for me. I think of the Estuary not far away with all the boats that my sister had shown me. That is it. That is what I must do. God will send a boat. Put my faith in God and the boat will be there.

So I try to disguise myself by tucking my long hair inside my jacket and sneak out of the hospital. So far, so good, I run and hide until I am sure I have got away. And then I start asking directions to Gillingham. I don't know how far it is but I was spurred on by the fact that I had to get there.

I reached the estuary and there they all were; many, many boats. How will I know which one it is? I must get to the water's edge and then I will know. So I start wading through the mud, it is getting deeper and deeper. I keep losing my shoes but I must carry on. Up to my waist in mud, it is very difficult to move. My shoes have broken and I have mud in my hair. I get as near to the

Cracking up & Barkin'

water as I can and look out toward the boats. The people on them are all watching me. How will I know which one of them God has sent? The voice in my head is telling me to get into the water and God will save me. God will show me. But the other voice is saying that I cannot swim and I will drown. I start to cry. My faith in God is not strong enough for me to get into the water. I cannot do this.

In a deep despair I turn around and head back towards land. But the mud is so deep and I am so very tired. I struggle through as far as I can and when I can go no further I see a man walking with a young girl. "Please help me" I shout.

"Just my luck" he said. But he waded through the mud and helped me reach dry land. I see the funfair there and manage to find the First Aid Tent.

"I have escaped from the mental hospital." They hosed me down with water as I am covered in mud and sit me in the tent to await the Police and my family.

So before I know it I am being escorted by my sister back to the hospital. I am so tired and despairing at my weakness.

I accept the futility of my situation and welcome the fact that I am to be put on medication. Anything to stop this from happening, I can't bear it any more.

Cracking up & Barkin'

I had sat up each night thinking I would be killed and it would look like suicide and now they were taking me into a side room, weighting me, measuring me, taking my blood pressure. I am facing execution, I thought. But I am so tired I just accept my situation.

They put me on largactil. I feel as though all the blood in my veins is being replaced by something toxic. The sensation in my legs is quite unbearable. And fairly soon, I feel that there is some kind of electrical beam coming down on my head. So I balance a pile of books on top of my bonce and concentrate on holding them there. This makes people laugh and my meds are replaced by haloperidol and something for the side effects. I even accept something to help me sleep.

I soon realise that this is a different type of nightmare. I cannot sit down. I cannot keep still. I pace up and down and from foot to foot. I spend my days walking up and down the building and my mind is no longer capable of cohesive thinking. They start to talk to me about where I am going to go.

I soon realise that if I am to escape this place I have to go back to my husband. So when he gets permission to take me and my son to McDonald's I go along. My son, sitting opposite, his little face wiring through an enormous burger when I find I have forgotten how to eat. I have a piece of food on my tongue but cannot work out how to bite it without biting my tongue. And on my return to the hospital my jaw got stuck and I could

Cracking up & Barkin'

not move my mouth. This is impossible; I must get off these drugs.

So I start to talk to the new young psychiatrist. She had said that she believed what had happened to me was a result of everything I had been through and when I said I was feeling better could she reduce the tablets she said that she would. From then on when I said I was feeling better I meant the side effects weren't so bad not that the thoughts had left me, although these were dampened. Another patient had told me not to tell the psychiatrists anything "I am psychic" she said, "the more you tell them the worse it will be". So I had learnt how to survive. If you told them anything they would increase the medication which was quite unbearable.

My psychiatrist was replaced by a retired Turkish psychiatrist. "Cannabis?" he said "I have not met anyone like you before; I want to get all of your family in here". Oh no, I thought, I'm not going to allow him to get his hands on my Mother and my son.

My husband asked permission to take me to London for the weekend. That is it, I thought, I must escape to London. Establish myself back in the flat, get my son back. So I escaped to London, my husband had arranged for my GP to put me under his care and I was made an appointment to attend daily at the Day Hospital of the nearest psychiatric hospital.

Cracking up & Barkin'

I met my new Psychiatrist. "Your problem is cannabis" she said "as long as you avoid it you will be fine". She started reducing my meds and telling me that as long as I remained drug free then my life would get back on track. But my fears were getting stronger. I knew what I believed that the fact that I no longer had any contact with cannabis seemed to make no difference. I was just relieved that the horrific side effects to the drugs were lessening. I had stood on the platform on the way home each night thinking of throwing myself in front of a train as I was incapable of any kind of life, incapable of caring for my young son. But I would tell myself that life might get better. I just had to escape from the system. And all I would hear from others was the dangers of cannabis "Ok" I thought, I'm avoiding cannabis but it makes no difference. But I had learnt to keep my thoughts to myself.

I managed to get discharged from the Day Hospital. What a relief that was. I had tried to while away the hours with nothing to do. They had offered art therapy and writing therapy so they could examine what was going on in my mind. But I didn't want that. My safety lay in them not knowing what was going on in my mind. And now I had escaped from the system I would act normal and they would leave me alone.

I settled back into life at home and for a little while it wasn't too bad. The ongoing nightmare of the medication was subsiding but as it did the realization that these terrible things really

Cracking up & Barkin'

were going on all around me increased. I felt that my thoughts were being listened to, I could hear the voices of others in my head talking to each other and decided the best thing to do was to sit and listen to them and work it out from there. And I must keep it to myself and avoid my husband who was watching me all the time. He had said if they wanted to give me electric shock treatment he would sign the papers. I moved back out of the bedroom.

I was trying to feed the three of us on the change I was given each morning. I could afford potatoes and eggs but aware if I ate my egg at lunch time I couldn't have it in the evening. I approached social security for money but was told that as I was married I could receive no money. If I was on my own with the child then they could help me. I was aware the bills weren't being paid and didn't know what to do.

And then I spoke with the social worker who visited the local community centre. "I know a good Solicitor" he said, "You can't carry on like this".

She was marvellous. A letter despatched to my husband asking him to leave the marital home and pay towards the bills until he did. And when he came home, I would climb out of the window, the quickest way into the garden, as I felt evil emanating from him whenever he approached.

Cracking up & Barkin'

Then the cavalry arrived. My friends hired a van and my husband and all his belongings were moved out. Philip remarked that "now Daddy has gone can I have a brother or sister". And on being told I couldn't manage that on my own he said "well wait till I grow up and I will help you". I laughed.

I got a job. I transferred the mortgage and everything else into my name. And it wasn't too bad for awhile. But I was becoming increasingly aware that my son was getting older and soon he would be at school and then he would be lost to me forever. My dreams of spending my days in his company would no longer be able to be realized and what of a brother or a sister for him?

I seemed to have quite a good relationship with my boss. We would talk about the powers and facet of the human mind. Many times I would sit and talk with him in his office, sometimes lunch with him. He would talk about his impending divorce and I would talk of mine. The years went by. Others in the Company had warned me that he could be artful, sly and cunning and to be careful. But I looked upon him as a kindly uncle; eccentric, but seemingly kind. And then one day he made a pass. So I stopped lunching in his office.

And that's when I started to see the other side of him. He would send me horrible notes. Accuse me of all sorts of things like making a mess in the kitchen. He started deducting my monthly trips to see the psychiatrist from my

Cracking up & Barkin'

holidays. I tried to keep going, kept my head down and got on with the work. And as the months went by he became nastier and nastier.

I no longer felt safe in the office from the fears I felt outside. He seemed to change from what I was seeing as an unpleasant man into somebody involved in the terrible crimes going on all around me. My work started to suffer. I could no longer remember how to do things. I would struggle in at weekends to try and correct the errors I had made during the week. I was so tired but told I was not due any holidays as I had used them up with my trips to the Psychiatrist and the school.

It was hard juggling a full-time job with running a home and bringing up a young child on my own and I was becoming increasingly upset by the fact that Philip was with others after school when he should have been with me. He was becoming increasingly difficult to manage and each night I had to buy him something on the way home or he refused to walk with me. Sometimes I would physically throw him over my shoulder and carry this seven year old kicking and punching me all the way home. By this time I was no longer sleeping nights and becoming more and more frightened by what I thought was going on all around me.

I had started to think that the eating of people was more widespread then I had previously thought. That the design of places like

Cracking up & Barkin'

spaghetti junction were designed to encourage as many traffic accidents as possible and that all the bodies, in reality, found their way into the sausages and the meat pies. That there was no such thing as vegetable fat, it was all human. Ham and pork... all human. And it wasn't just going on here... it was all the pure descendants of the Saxons. That's the big secret of the Freemasons; that's what the army, the secret services, the fascist parties are really all about.

The voices in my head, they were coming from an invisible electronic beam attached to the satellites. That's what they were really doing. And it wasn't just here; it was all over the western world. Just to produce as much human meat as possible and anyone who found out, it would happen to them. So I couldn't tell anybody what I had discovered as it would lead to this or sudden death.

Then, one Friday lunchtime, my Social Worker arrived with another at my office, put me in the car and carted me off to be sectioned. It was half -term and Philip was staying with his Granny in Kent. "You've been smoking cannabis again" she said. It was true that I had smoked the occasional joint over the years. I was so tired with the continuous voices in my head both day and night and so frightened by what I had thought was going on that it stopped me from sleeping. Many nights I had spent sitting guard outside Philip's bedroom all night clutching a hammer and then back to work the next day. I couldn't let these evil people get their hands on my son.

'Right" she said as she signed the papers to section me. "I want to put you on depot injections (regular injections of strong antipsychotic drugs) or you will lose Philip". I had always feared these injections as they seemed to induce some kind of brain damage in those receiving them but I had no choice.

I was made to lie on the bed with my trousers around my ankles whilst they injected me in the bum. I was to be given a weekly injection to start with and then fortnightly. The anti-psychotic is in oil which seeps into the system gradually which is much stronger than the tablets as it goes directly to the brain instead of through the stomach. I could no longer bear the side effects, could no longer keep still. I was pacing up and down, my legs becoming more and more tired. I told my psychiatrist that it was unbearable; she remarked that I was suffering cannabis withdrawal. I tried to ask if sleep deprivation had caused all of this and she snapped "I've told you it's the cannabis"

I was discharged from the hospital and went back to work but my mind was becoming cloudier by the day and I could no longer concentrate on what I was supposed to do. And I started to put on weight, a lot of weight. Eventually, I realised that I was incapable of logical thinking, my mind was empty. I would just pace from foot to foot or up and down the hall for hours. If I managed to sit I would rock back and forth uncontrollably. This was a living hell. I was told to take it a day at a time and get on with my life. But for me, I was living it a minute at a time – there seemed to be no end to this excruciating nightmare. I could no longer work; no longer pay the mortgage or the bills. What was I to do?

So Philip and I sold up and moved to Norwich to be near my parents and my sister who were also moving there. This way I could pay off my mortgage and move to a cheaper house. And then I could manage on my benefits.

I hadn't been in Norwich long when my new psychiatrist sorted out a new side-effect tablet. What a relief. I could sit down and although I still rocked back and forth uncontrollable, at least I could stay seated.

He was a kindly man and told me not to be frightened, I was totally safe, and he would look after me. He put me on tablets as well as the depot injections. I quickly went from the 7 stone a few months before up to 16 stone as the medication slows down the metabolism. And my mind could no longer retain anything. I could no longer read. I could no longer think through any problem. When asked a question my mind was completely blank, completely empty, as though somebody had pulled a black blind down over it. I would listen to other people on the bus chatting to one another; I would witness my sisters at family gatherings catching up with each other's lives and

Cracking up & Barkin'

long to be able to do that.

The years went by, other people having lives, my son Philip bringing himself up. Any problem, anything that had to be done like replacing the washing machine Philip had to negotiate and I would stand there, pacing from foot to foot, incapable to doing anything. I sat rocking on the sofa for the best part of 13 years. I still felt fear sometimes when I went outside. Still felt that evil things were going on around me but I was relatively safe in my little terrace house in the middle of many similar terraces.

And then I met my last psychiatrist. "Very pleased to meet you" he said, as he shook my hand. We went into his room and he asked "what would you like me to do for you?"

I said that I would like to come off the depot injections (after all Philip was an adult now and could no longer be put into care), that I didn't want to spend another 13 years rocking on the sofa. I had lost all those years and I wanted my life back. So he looked into it, increased my tablets and stopped the injections. I started to wake up a little, aware of what was going on around me. I started to trust this psychiatrist. I told him I had never agreed with the reason given for my illness and if I wrote down in brief what I had been going through at the time of my first breakdown would he read it.

So for the first time in 20 years I felt able to confide in somebody, not frightened that I would be shunned for speaking my mind. Trusting a psychiatrist was something new to me. I put down my thoughts and posted them and on my next visit he said that he believed that cannabis was not the reason for my psychosis. He believed that I would have been ill with or without my former nightcap.

He had read of the deep emotion I had felt at being separated from Philip. The guilt I had felt at being unable to breast feed my premature infant and then being forced to go back to full-time work when he was only two. He said that the one thing he has found common amongst schizophrenics was that they were all heartbroken.

I started looking forward to my appointments and he not only guided me through my thoughts and worries but also helped me with the arthritis which I had developed through gaining so much weight. Another side effect of the medication was that my periods had stopped resulting in premature osteoporosis which runs in the family anyway.

Then, at my request, he gradually, over the years reduced the amount of tablets I had to take. I very slowly started to wake up. The tendency to rock back and forth or pace about seemed more controllable most of the time. I started to lose weight. I also realised that the voices I used to hear were now replaced by my own voice, the one everybody hears when they are thinking, within the same place in my brain.

Cracking up & Barkin'

He helped me cope with my Mother who had developed dementia and any troubles I had with my son. He was a very important part of my life.

And then, a year ago, he moved on. His replacement who has never seen me, will only see me if I am in crisis. My Mother and sister have both left Norwich. And then my son moved to Cambridge... So I am left alone with my fears. I am usually able to reason with myself when frightened with what might be going on outside. If not, I have been empowered to increase my own meds until I feel a little better.

I am now able to understand where a lot of my fears have come from. The electronic beams and the cannibalism come from a record I was listening to. The witchcraft and Satanism from all those Dennis Wheatley books I read when still quite young. The feeling that I am being watched, is that anything to do with my early belief that God was watching me wherever I went, that my Guardian Angel was writing down whatever I thought or did and on Judgement Day If I didn't pass the test, I would burn for all eternity in the fires of hell. That my son, who remains un-christened, will never go to Heaven, but to a place called Limbo? I try to reason with myself that these thing are purely fiction, written my man to control man, that the fact I don't go to Church, that I instigated a divorce, that I don't believe in God will not result in an indefinite visit to Satan's hell-hole.

Cracking up & Barkin'

I tell myself that the fact I have put all these things down on paper for others to see will not result in the evil ones coming after me again. I have sat in my bedroom blanking my mind so they won't hear me thinking. Any kind of stress and I am pacing up and down like a caged animal aware that others are trying to believe I am back to normal.

As for the cannabis, I am not saying that the heavy use of cannabis, particularly the stronger strains available these days especially on the young cannot result in schizophrenia, it clearly can. What I am saying is that the trauma experienced before and during an episode should not be dismissed or belittled purely because they had shared a spliff or two at the end of the day .

I believe that my psychosis was pre-empted by a form of post-traumatic stress disorder but find that now I have woken up I have no professional help in working through the remaining trauma.

As for the fear and guilt taught by the church and put into my subconscious from any early age, I despair that these things are still being taught to our young. And as much as I reason with myself, I still feel frightened when going past a church.

And schizophrenics, many deserve a bravery medal.

I have sat over the months writing this,

Cracking up & Barkin'

sometimes crying for the years I have lost and for my son, some times frightened that I will be mentally invaded and hunted by those who would harm me and can only hope that these writings will help others who are like me or who seek to understand.

Cracking up & Barkin'

Barkin'

Short Stories from the World of Psychosis

Deirdre Geraghty

Cracking up & Barkin'

Cracking up & Barkin'

To my family

Cracking up & Barkin'

Cracking up & Barkin'

CONTENTS

Wix's Lane

The journey home

Car number plates

Reporting a crime

Trip to Corsham

A friendly satellite

Seeing red

Insurance

Fruzsina

Friends above

The scream within me

Warminster

Trip to the Doctors

Murder in the flats

The Joker

The Dome

Cracking up & Barkin'

Cracking up & Barkin'

Wix's Lane

I had pondered long and hard on what was happening to me, wondering if it had something to do with where I lived in Wix's Lane, Clapham Common. Wix was another name for witch. I tried to believe, as I had been told, it had been named after Charles Wix, a builder, but my mind kept coming back to the thought that there was something special about this place.

I searched for older and older maps and then came across one dated 1827. There wasn't much here in those days just Wix's Lane, Mount Nod opposite and The Chase.

Wanting to know more I tried to discover anything I could about Mount Nod. It seemed to be situated in what is now the grounds of a monastery. That seemed relevant in itself as many of our religious buildings were built on pagan sites. Try as I did, I could find no information about this place.

And the Chase, why was it so named?

My mind came back to Wix's Lane. Perhaps it was special. I see that there are a few buildings on the Lane, one of them on the site of my house. Perhaps it had something to do with this house? Perhaps what was happening to me, this sensitivity that others around me do not have, this awareness of what is going on around me that I never had before, has something to do with this

Cracking up & Barkin'

place. Maybe it has happened to others who have lived here before me. In times gone past maybe I would have been called a witch.

      I pictured people gathering on The Chase in times gone past. What or who did they chase? And what happened at Mount Nod opposite. I started to be filled with a fear that the person living on this spot was the prey and hauled off to Mount Nod for some form of ritual. Perhaps it is a place where witches were burnt.

      Filled with a fear that there are still those who would gather in the Chase and they would be after me.

      I tried to look in the grounds of the monastery for a sight of Mount Nod but to no avail. I tried to calm myself with the thought that nothing sinister could go on there now. My mind constantly coming back to the vision of myself hauled off to some unimaginable event.

      I spent many nights sitting through the darkness, clutching a hammer, fearing those who might be creeping up the Lane, relieved by the fact that nobody would stop me.

Cracking up & Barkin'

The journey home

Meeting him in the evening was the highlight of my day. Philip, a golden child, blessed with a special quality of hidden depths. We would make daisy chains along the way, as a stretch of Clapham Common lay between the Nursery and the house.

Past the church and onwards towards the swings and the bandstand. I would jump and skip and run and tell him to do the same. I felt free on this large expanse of green with it's trees dotted here and there and I laughed and skipped and felt the wind in my hair. Philip, alongside, laughing as he ran.

I looked up towards the tops of the trees and up beyond to where the satellites stood. They could do such good up there above the clouds. "Come on" I said "let's shout at them". I heard my voice, at first friendly, encouraging them to do their best and then getting angrier for I feared they would do their worst. I encouraged Philip to do the same but he never did.

Cracking up & Barkin'

Cracking up & Barkin'

Car number plates

For quite some time now my eyes have been drawn to car number plates. As though they have some significance in all of this. I would look at the numbers and decide if they were good numbers or bad and how they reflected on each car's owner.

     I see on the news that the satellites can photograph the car number plates from way up there. When it suddenly dawns on me. That's what I have been doing. They have been picturing the cars' plates through my eyes, along an electronic beam attached to the top of my head.

     So, as I venture out, I scan each and every number plate as I pass by. Glad to help.

Cracking up & Barkin'

Reporting a crime

"Can I report a crime that hasn't happened yet?" I said to the Policeman "The people down the road are going to kill me". "You mean bogeymen?" he said. "No, they are real people, I would just feel safer if you knew". "Right" he said, "I'll write it down".

Cracking up & Barkin'

Cracking up & Barkin'

Trip to Corsham

Safe in the understanding that if I did everything in a clockwise fashion only good would happen. I would go to the corner shop the long way round in order to bring good luck on those who lived within.

My plans to visit Corsham were a little worrying. I checked the map. It certainly wouldn't be in a clockwise direction. I tried to put my fears aside and we set off for Victoria Coach Station. I checked the Bay Number when I bought the ticket and checked again with the driver when we boarded the coach. "Yes, I'll put you off at Corsham" he said.

My friend Jean had given me instructions on what to do on our arrival at 1.00 and she would have lunch waiting.

We were quite excited on the journey and, right on time, the driver shouted "Corsham" and put us off. Taking Philip by the hand I looked about us. But instead of the country lane I see a busy road and a fly-over. Then I see a building quite close by. "What are the Royal Hampshire Constabulary doing in Wiltshire" I said to Philip. We ventured into the building where I promptly announce that I think we are lost. Both of the policemen smile kindly and tell us we are in Cosham (pronounced Corsham) in Hampshire. "It quite often happens".

Aware that I only have a ticket home and

the tube fair I wonder what to do. They show me a map, we are a long way from Wiltshire and I picture Jean waiting with our lunch down a quiet lane.

"Never mind" they said "we will see what we can do". One of them disappears into the back and, on his return, he puts us in his police car and takes us to the local bus station, delivering us safely into the hands of the Station Manager. All arrangements have been made and we are taken to the canteen and bought a sandwich and a drink. Then we are handed over to the driver of the coach to Portsmouth. A little while later we are met by another Station Manager and the driver of the coach to Bath. "Yes" he said, "You have just enough time to look at the ships before you climb on board".

Many hours later we arrive in Bath to be met by yet another Station Manager and Jean who are there to greet us.

"Thank heavens for the Royal Hampshire Constabulary" I think to myself and then chuckle at the fact we have arrived in a clockwise direction. Is somebody trying to tell me something?

A friendly satellite

Looking out from the garden room into the night sky I watch the stars. There is something very peaceful at this time of night and I feel a sense of calm.

One of the stars, much brighter than the rest seems to move quite a way to the right and then back again. I realise it is a satellite saying "hello" in the only way they can and their way of proving to me that my thoughts are real. I watch for quite awhile as they dart back and forth across the night sky before I head for bed.

Awaking early, I nip out quickly to the shop for cigarettes. I look up to the sky. And there before me, the most beautiful rainbow, much wider than a normal one, which disappears into a cloud but mysteriously stops there. I look around and there is nobody about.

The guys in the satellites have created it just for me, an absolute copy of the painting on the side of my favourite Greenpeace mug. They would much prefer to be creating the weather, all the good they could do, instead of driving people mad with their electronic beams.

I hurry home.

Cracking up & Barkin'

Cracking up & Barkin'

Seeing red

As though seeing things for the first time, I realise the red objects in the house look like a trail of blood from the back door. I gather them all up and leave them outside before i go to bed.

Cracking up & Barkin'

Insurance

Gripped in the knowledge that I am to be murdered in the night I 'phone a friend. "I am writing their names upon the wall" I tell her, "that is my insurance". One by one their names come to me and I write them upon the wall, firstly in permanent red ink and then in lipstick. I know they can see what I am doing and wont be able to harm me whilst their names are on the wall.

Cracking up & Barkin'

Fruzsina

Fruzsina, my friend for many years has come to help. Always there when I need her she cares for Philip whilst I fight my demons in the bedroom beyond. She was from Transylvania which I always thought was a fictional place until I met her. And then, when I had known her many years, I discovered she was a Countess.

She came into the room to try and help. I always felt reassured when she was there and she asked what she could do. I looked at her closely and then saw her canines had grown unusually long. "She really is a vampire" I thought. I wasn't frightened. It was somehow very reassuring to have a vampire on my side. I thought about the fact that she was a vegetarian and chuckled at my assumption that she gained her protein from all that blood.

She went home and I found that I was being lifted into a seated position by hands from behind me. I knew there was nobody there but felt the hands of three or four peopled kneeling behind me on the bed. I looked at the wall opposite and saw pictures moving on the plain white wall. As though somebody was showing a film show from a projector behind me.

Those behind were whispering that I have to fight my corner, their hands holding me firm. I see all sorts of creatures threatening me from the wall beyond. Bats, lions, bears and snakes all

Cracking up & Barkin'

coming at me one after another. I have to fight them off with the power of my mind or they will destroy me.

    Eventually, I can fight no longer and I collapse in a heap upon the bed.

Friends above

It's a bright sunny day and I strike out in flimsy clothes to get supplies. It is a happy day and I grin to myself as I meander down the Lane.

Suddenly, as if from nowhere, the skies open and the rain falls heavily to the ground. Those around me run for cover but I remain perfectly dry as I walk along the Lane. The guys in the satellites are raining on everyone else but me and I chuckle to myself. I feel very special.

Cracking up & Barkin'

Cracking up & Barkin'

The scream within me

Having spent a few days in Battersea where I could feel safe and get some sleep, we travelled home. David, my friend, took us the short distance by car and left us at the front door.

I turned the key. It was all in darkness. I slowly crept towards the light switch which was halfway down the hall. I felt a presence in the house which seemed to be coming towards me, nearer and nearer. I heard a loud and prolonged scream and realised, with shock, that it was coming from deep within me.

David returned and turned the light on and I ventured inside aware that I had always thought myself too inhibited to scream.

Cracking up & Barkin'

Warminster

Glancing at my watch to see how long till my next cigarette, I pop another sweet in my mouth and, again, look out the window. The coach speeds along the road towards Bath and I stare out trying to while away the time. Everything had been going well and I was pacing myself until I could again feed my nicotine addiction.

I start to feel a little strange and then I am gripped by an unknown fear. We are going through a town and I am aware that I don't like this place. The fear growing within me. I look out to discover we are in Warminster.

What it is about this place I do not know but I will feel much happier when we have left it far behind. I wonder why it is called 'Warminster'.

I mention this to my friends on our arrival and am told "Warminster has more UFO sightings than any other place in the country".

Cracking up & Barkin'

Trip to the Doctors

"Hello, come in, sit down" he said at the doorway. Dr. Dunwoody was a kindly man and I felt safe in his hands. I was careful not to let anything slip for if he knew what I know this would happen to him.

I walked home hoping he would be okay and looked at the time. End of surgery. I knew there was a lot of traffic on the road and started to feel he was in terrible danger. Somebody was trying to run him off the road. Perhaps I had let something slip after all. If I concentrate very hard perhaps I can will him safely home. This is a warning and I must be doubly vigilant in the future.

Cracking up & Barkin'

Cracking up & Barkin'

Murder in the flats

We had taken a short cut through the council flats on our way home. I had never been this way before. There was a large tank situated in the middle surrounded by security railings and I wondered what it was. There was nobody about and I wondered where everybody was.

Here in the safety of my own home I had a terrible thought. What if all the people were dead? All gassed in their own homes in the middle of the night. Who would know? Their bodies destroyed in that tank of acid.

I had noticed that many of the flats were boarded up. I would keep away from there.

Cracking up & Barkin'

The Joker

I was very pleased with the nursery. The walls painted white with it's large alphabet and red and white gingham curtains. The details in the room was painted green. I had always like red and green together.

Suddenly, gripped in the belief that red and green are the Joker's colours, I rush to the shop to buy a tin of yellow. Hurriedly, I paint over all the green.

Cracking up & Barkin'

Cracking up & Barkin'

The Dome

Enclosed in a see-through dome, like something from a science fiction, it felt wonderfully safe. I didn't know where it had come from but everything within it was still and quiet and safe. It seemed to go the length of the Lane and I was near the centre.

I sat in the sitting room. It was dark outside and the grubby glass of the window had somehow disappeared. It was as if the bush outside was practically in the room. All was still and altogether magical.